AF489233

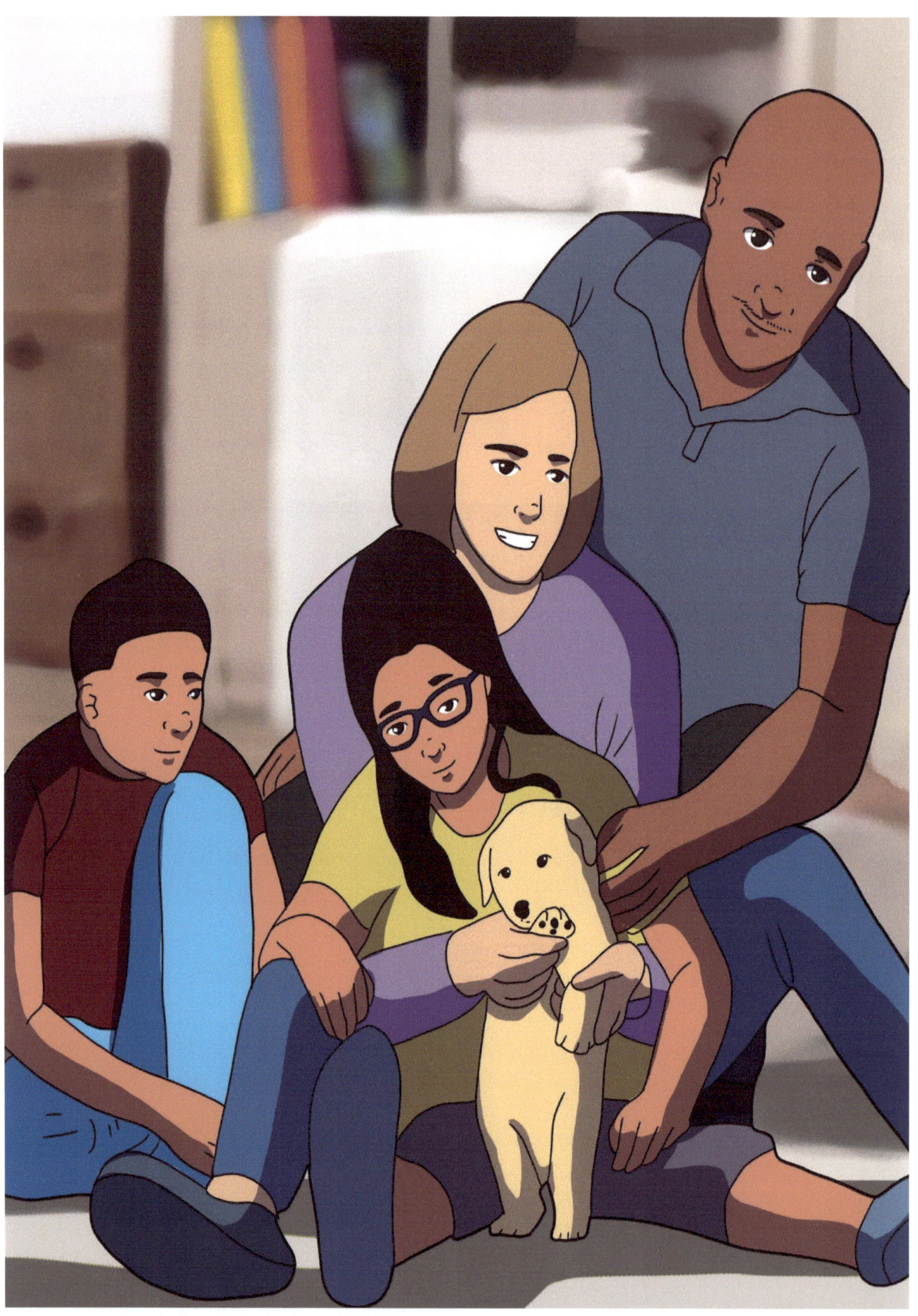

Meet Aliyah and Kyron.

We call them Ali and Ky.

Ali and Ky live with their Mom, Dad,

and their dog Bruno.

The family loves spending time

together and will soon find they will

be spending even more time together.

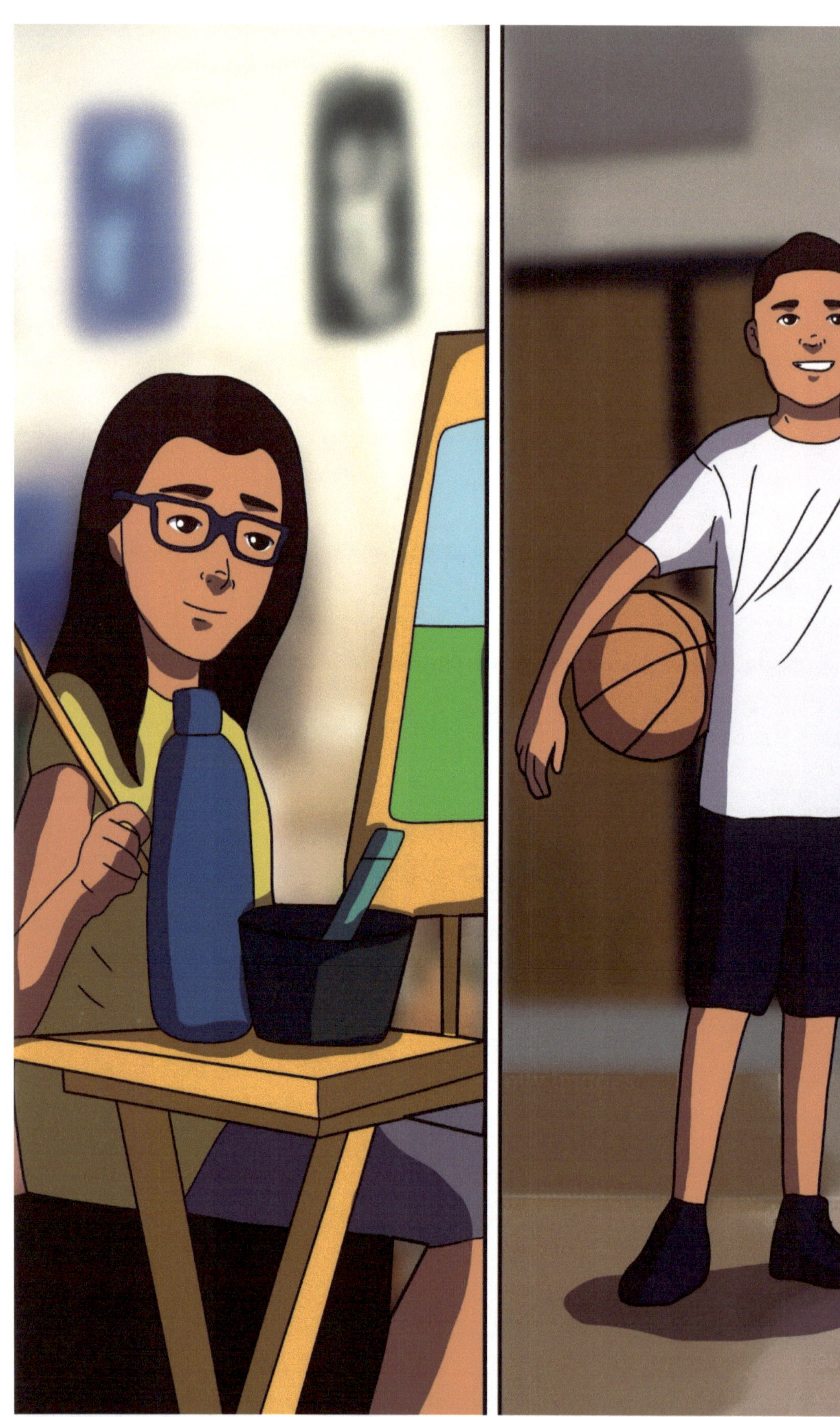

Ali and Ky enjoy going to school,
where they get to learn about new
things, and see their friends and
teachers.

Ali's favorite classes are
Art and Music.

Ky's favorite classes are
Reading and Gym

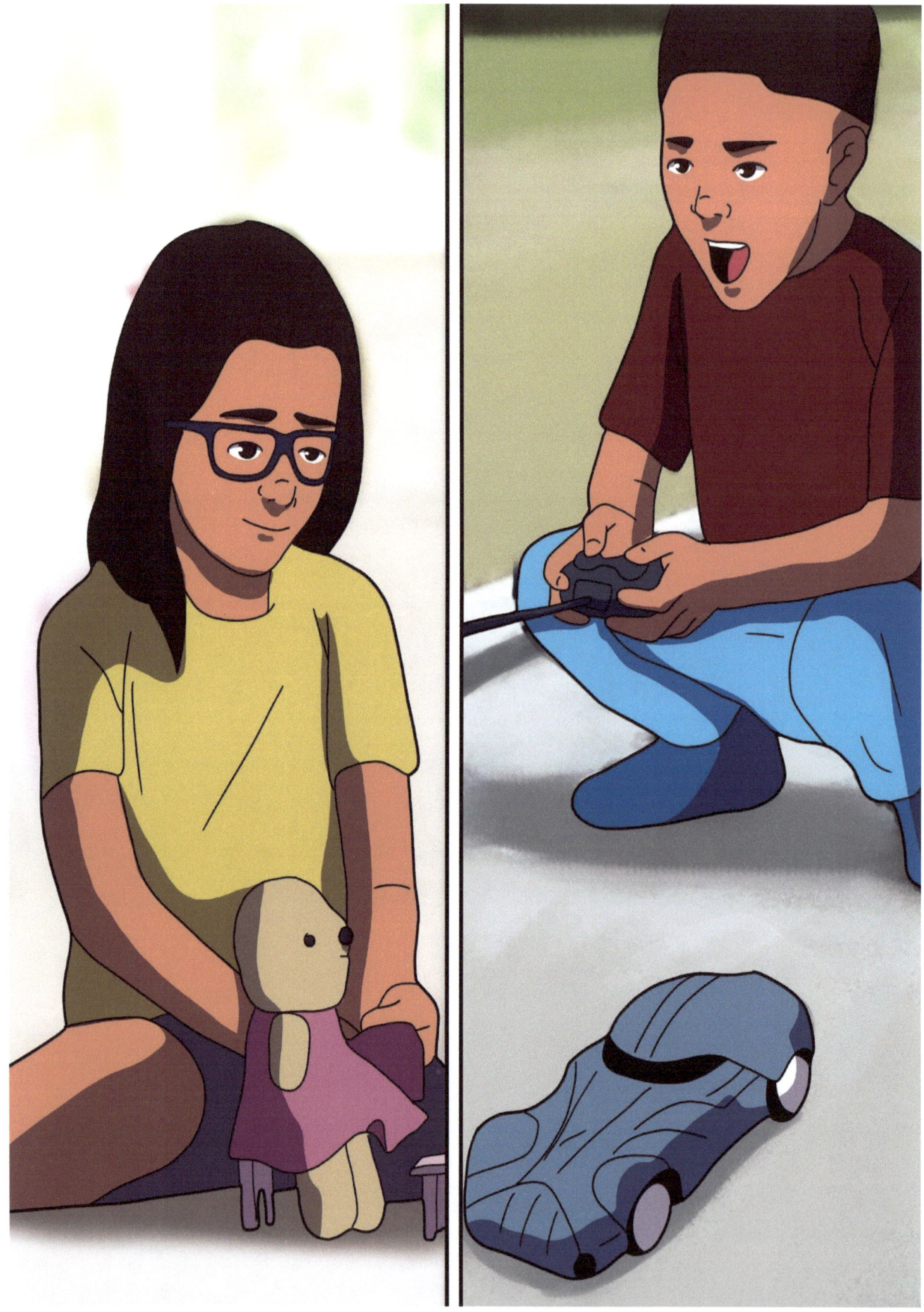

After school, Ali and Ky like to play
with their friends, ride bikes,
scooters, and play on their hover
boards.

Ky likes to play basketball and drive
remote control racing cars with his
friends.

Ali loves playing dolls, dress up, and
any pretend games that require her
and her friends to use their
imagination.

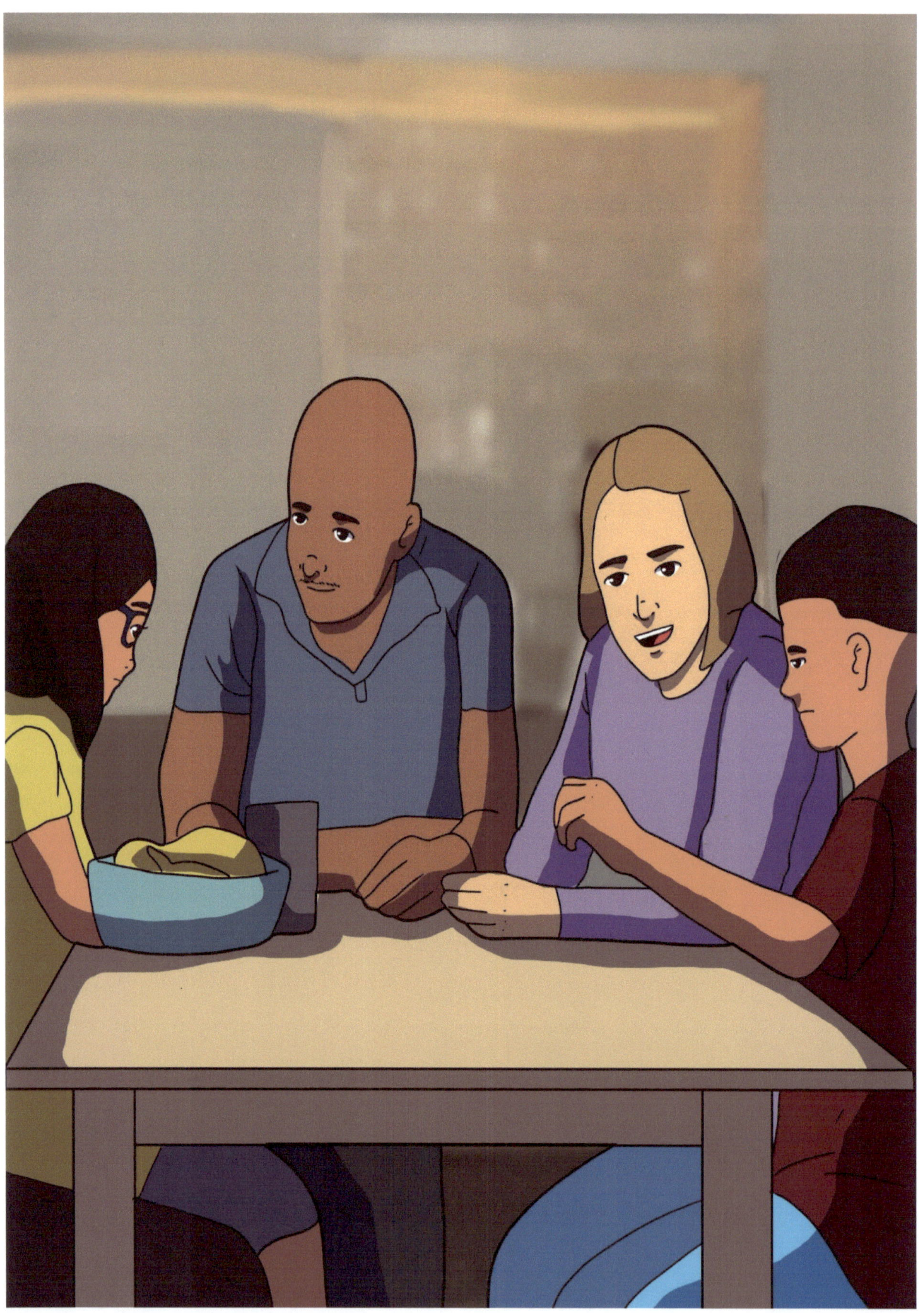

Today is a different day as Mom and Dad sit Ali and Ky down to tell them they will not be going to school this morning. "Why?" ask Ali and Ky.

"Dad and I will be working from home and the two of you will homeschool for the next few weeks to quarantine from COVID-19 (Coronavirus)" says Mom.

"What is the Coronavirus?" asks Ali. "What does quarantine mean?" asks Ky.

"The Coronavirus is a very contagious illness that has been causing people all over the world to become very sick. It can cause you to cough, have a fever, and in some cases make it hard to breathe," says Dad.

"Quarantine means to separate from others for a specific time until it is safe for everyone to be together again," says Mom.

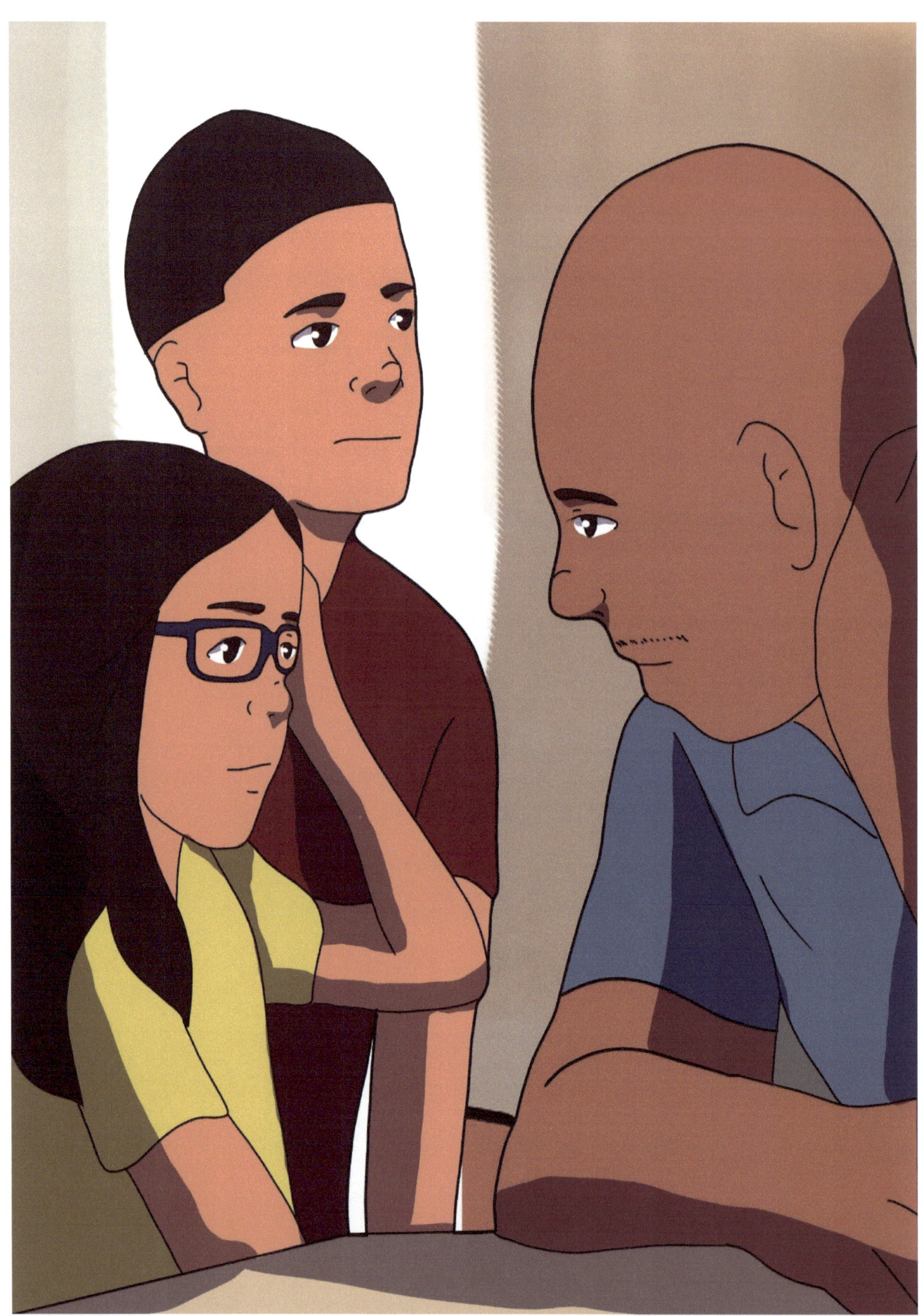

"I don't want to get the Coronavirus,"
says Ali, feeling scared.

"I don't want to get the Coronavirus
either," agrees Ky.

Dad speaks to the kids about the
importance of following the rules and
doing their best to stay safe during
the coronavirus quarantine.

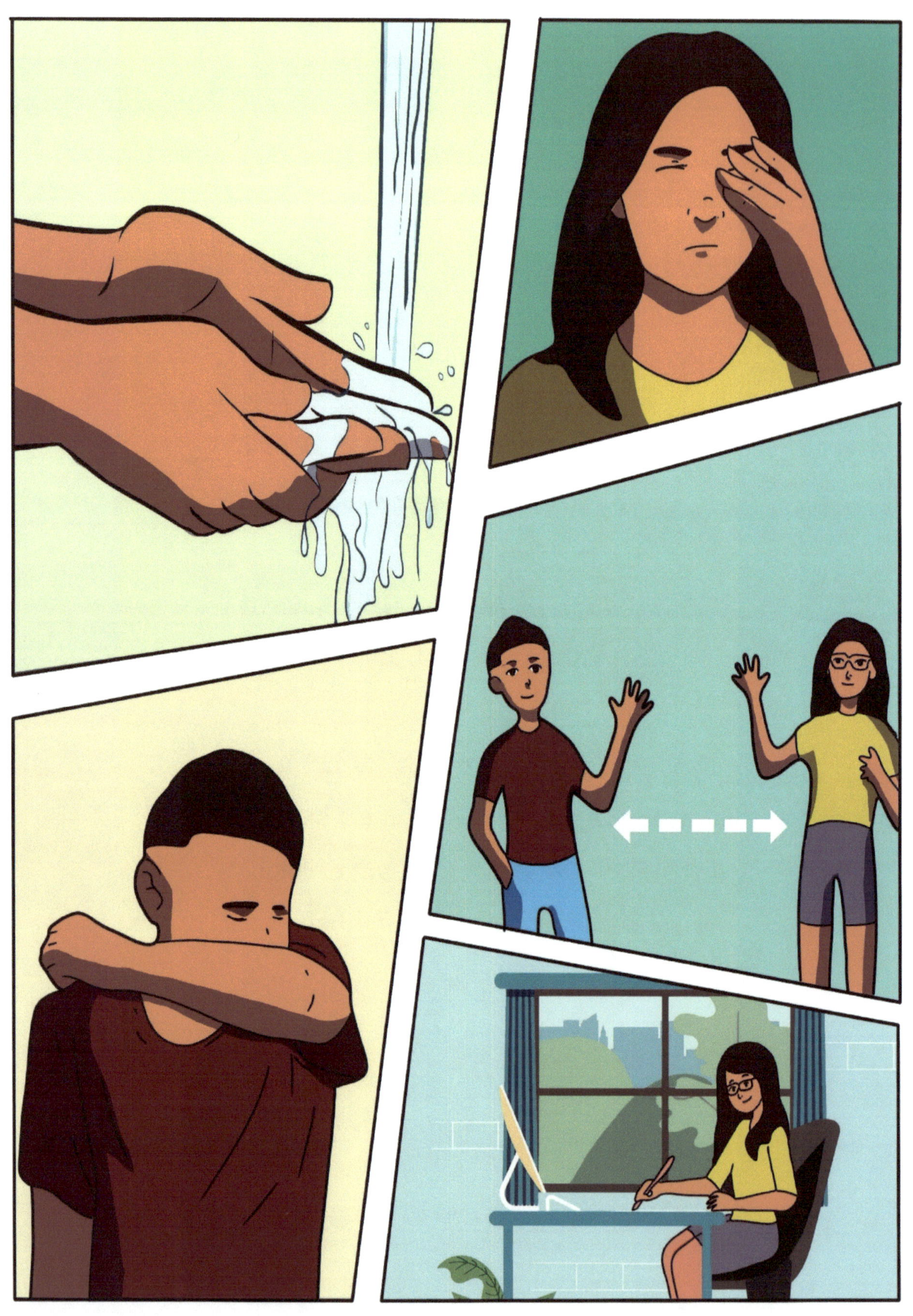

You can protect yourself from
spreading the Coronavirus by doing
these key things on a regular basis"
says Dad.

Wear a mask when out in public places

Wash your hands as often as possible

Cough into your elbow

Avoid touching your face

Avoid close contact with others

Stay home if you can

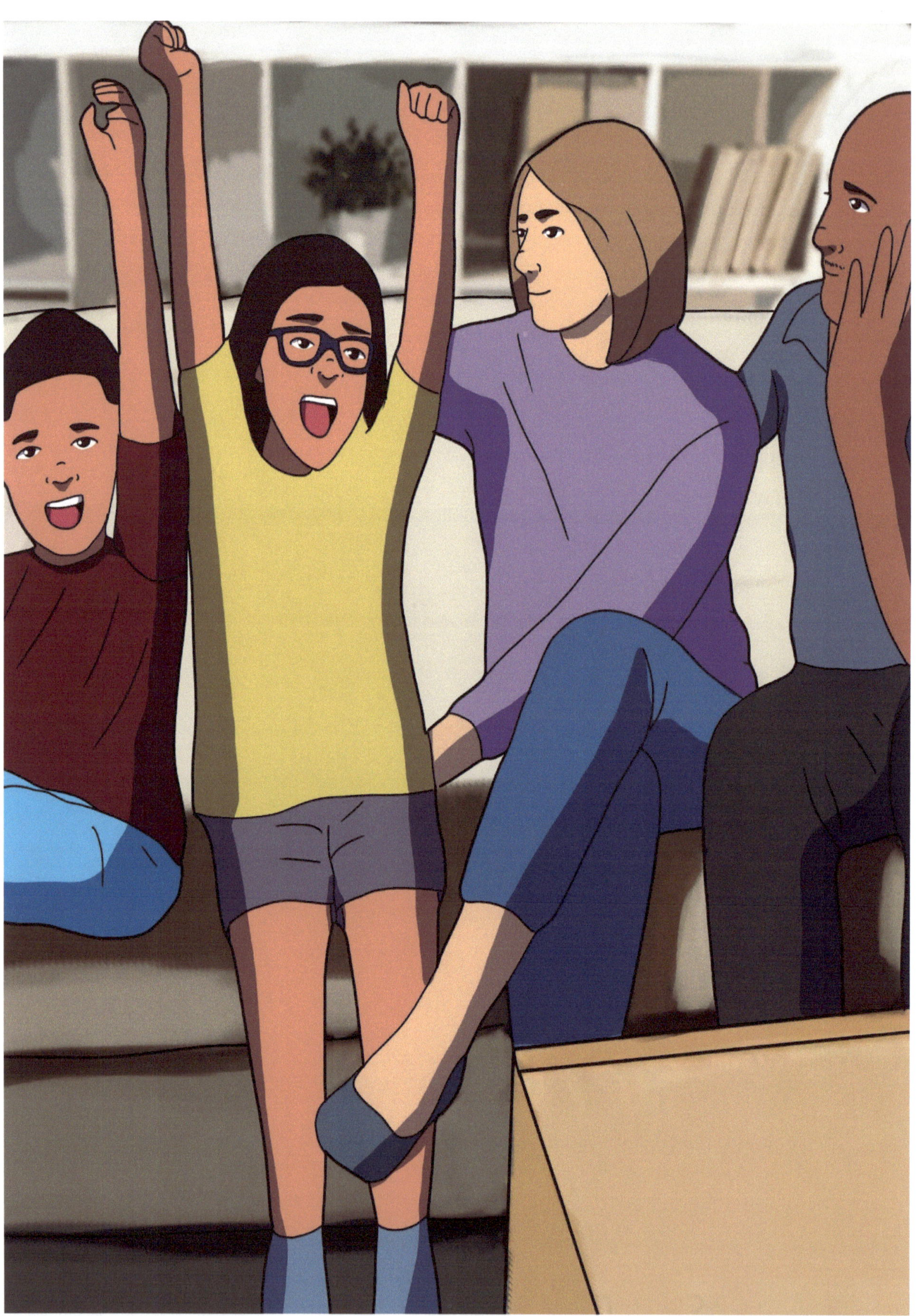

Ali and Ky have many questions.

"Does this mean we can actually stay home from school?" asks Ali. "Hooray, no school!" cheers Ky.

"Yes, this means you will be staying home from school, but you will still have to complete your daily school assignments," replies Mom.

"Can we have a sleepover?" asks Ali.

"No, quarantine means we have to stay a safe distance away from family and friends until it is safe to be together." says Mom.

"Can we still go on vacation?" asks Ky.

"No, it is recommended that we do not travel until the virus is under control to prevent it from spreading" says Dad.

"It doesn't seem like we can do anything, "grumble Ali and Ky.

"Don't worry, we will figure out a way to get through this and have fun as a family," says Dad.

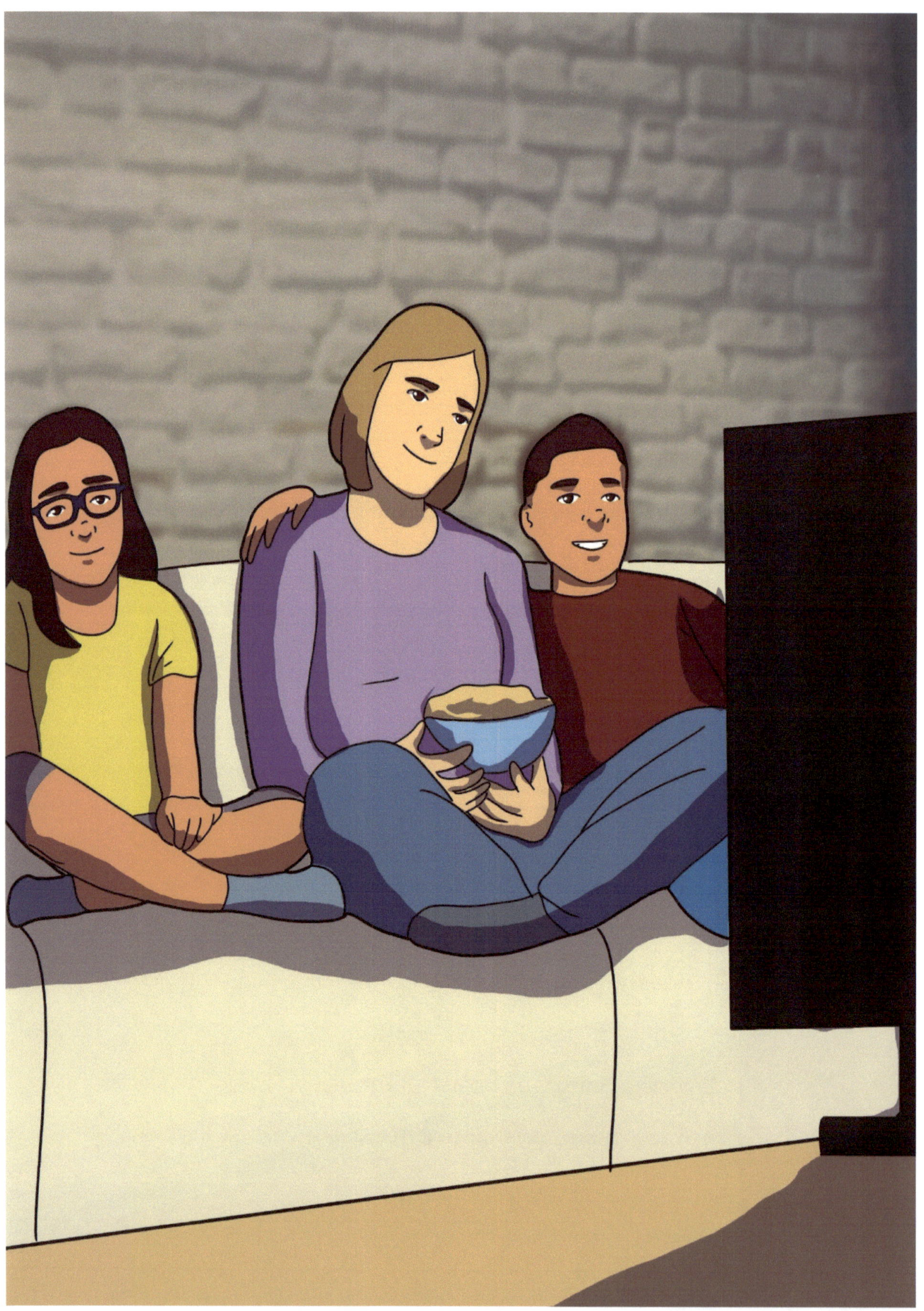

After a few days of being at home,
Ali and Ky start to get bored.

"Mom, can we go to the movies?" asks
Ali.

"Yeah, I'm bored!" complains Ky.

"There is plenty to do" says Mom.

"We can watch a movie, do puzzles,
draw, and color pictures," suggests
Mom.

Ali and Ky loved to watch movies, do
puzzles, and color pictures.

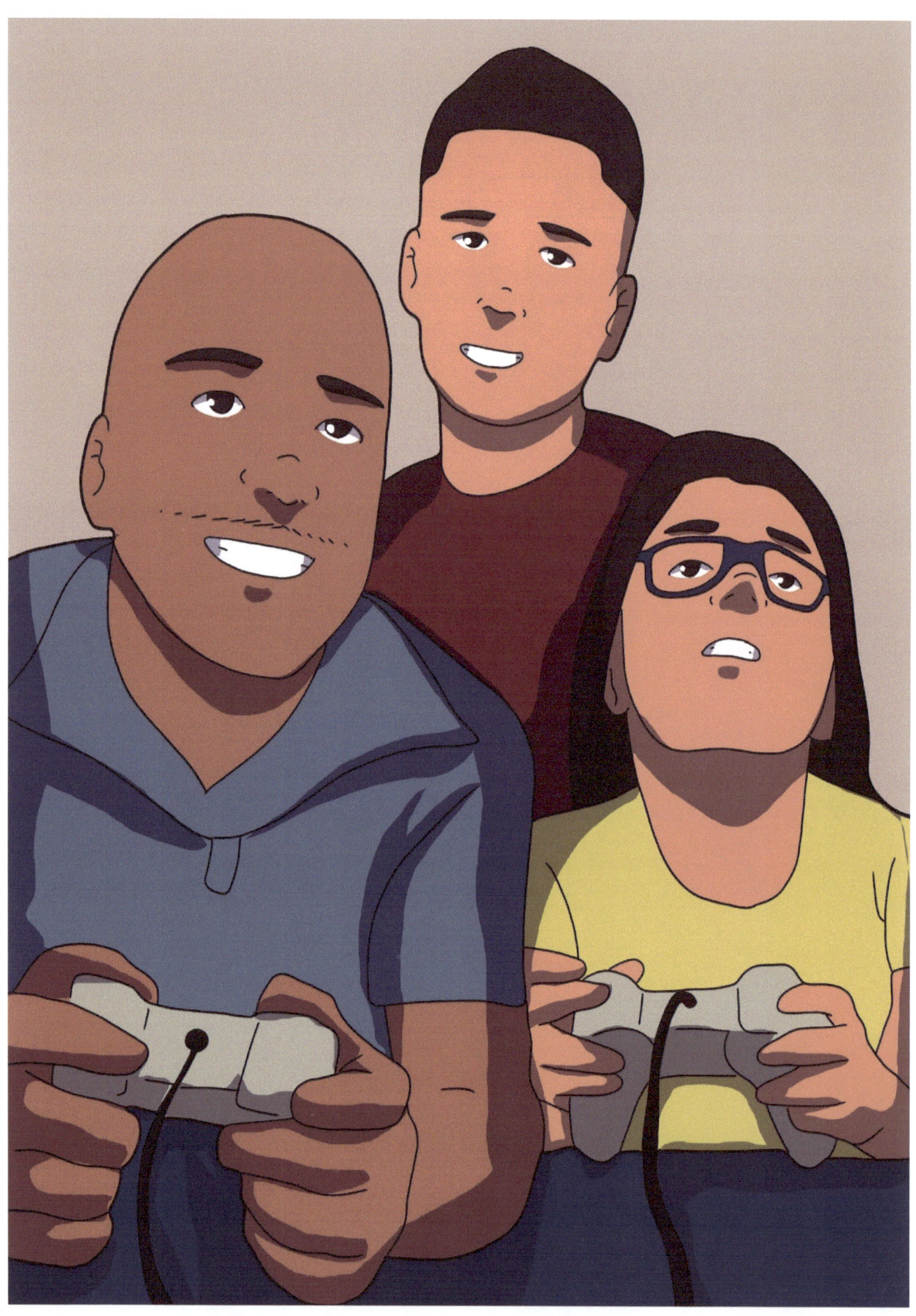

The next day Ali asked, "Dad, can we go bowling?"

"Yeah, I'm bored, there is nothing to do," says Ky.

"There is plenty to do" says Dad.

"We can play video games and race cars," offers Dad.

Ali and Ky love playing video games and racing cars.

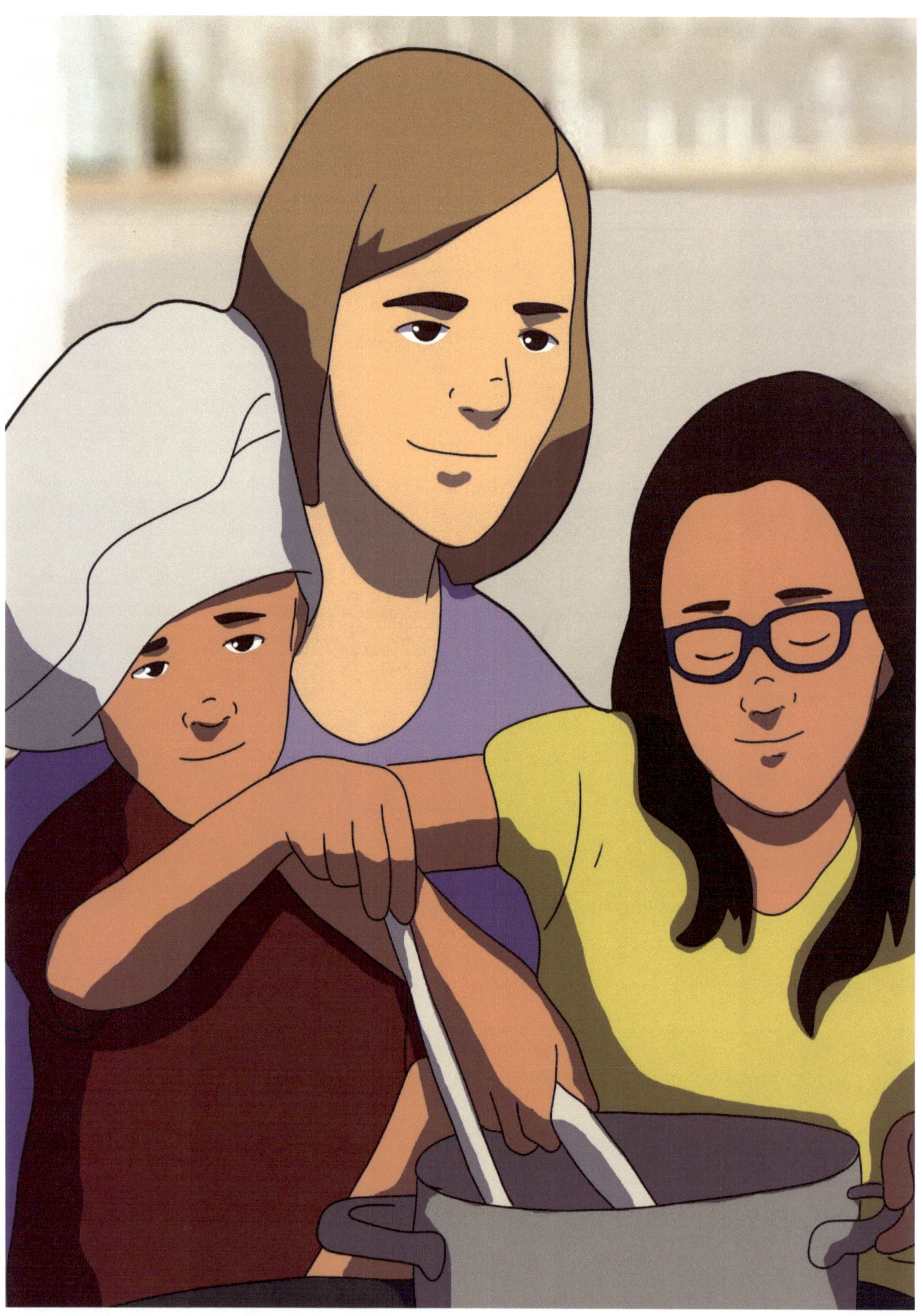

The next day, "Mom, can we go out to eat?" asks Ali.

"Yeah, I'm bored, there is nothing to do," says Ky.

"There is plenty to do" says Mom.

"The two of you can help me make dinner tonight, we can bake cookies for dessert, and watch a family movie," says Mom.

Ali and Ky love to help make dinner, bake cookies, and watch a family movie.

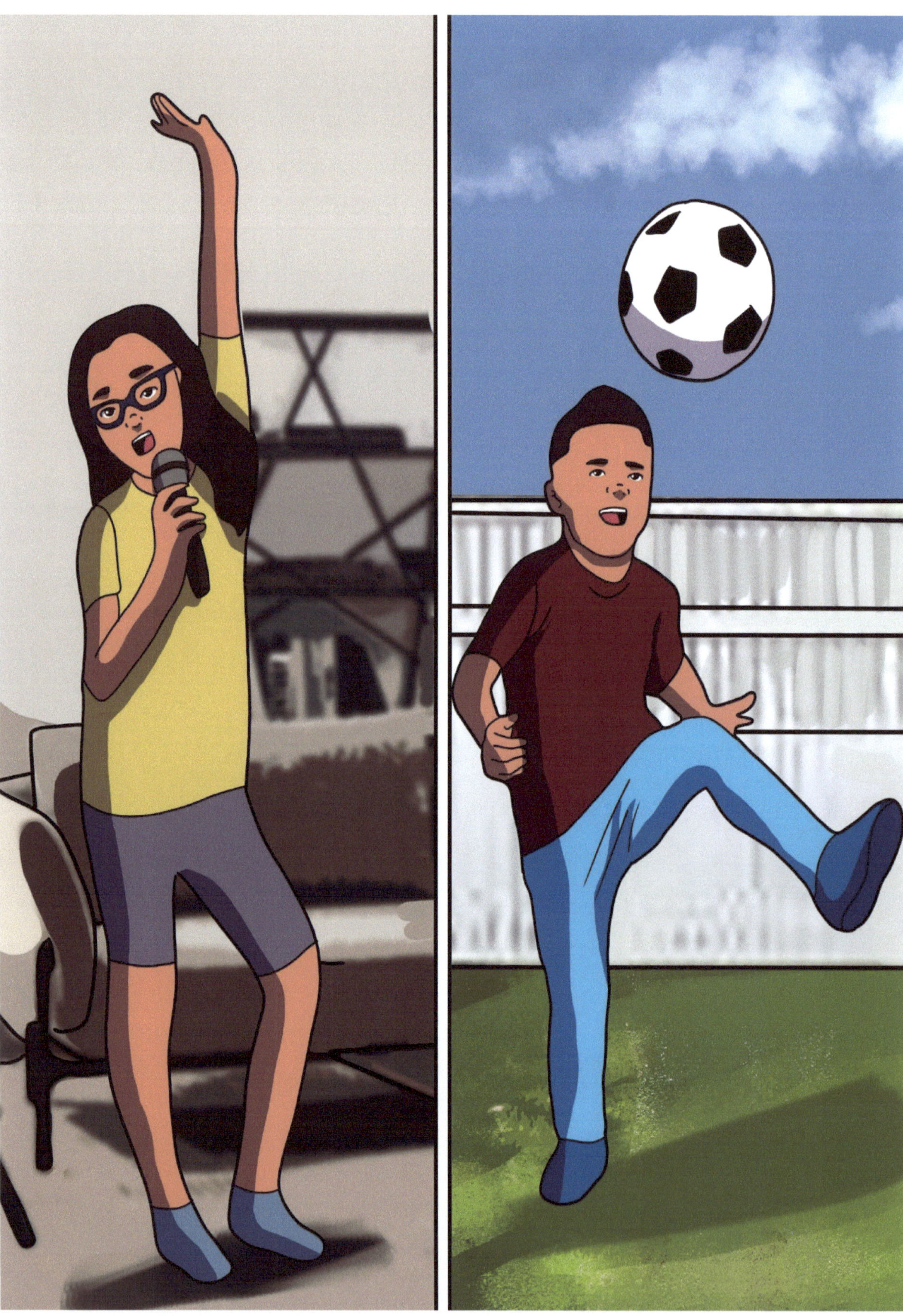

The next day, "Dad can I go to my
singing class?" asks Ali.

"Dad, can I go to basketball practice?"
asks Ky.

"Yeah, we are bored, there is nothing
to do," say Ali and Ky.

"There is plenty to do" says Dad.

"We can play basketball, soccer,
hockey, or baseball outside.
We can have a karaoke singing
contest," adds Dad.

Ali and Ky love to play sports outside,
and have singing contests.

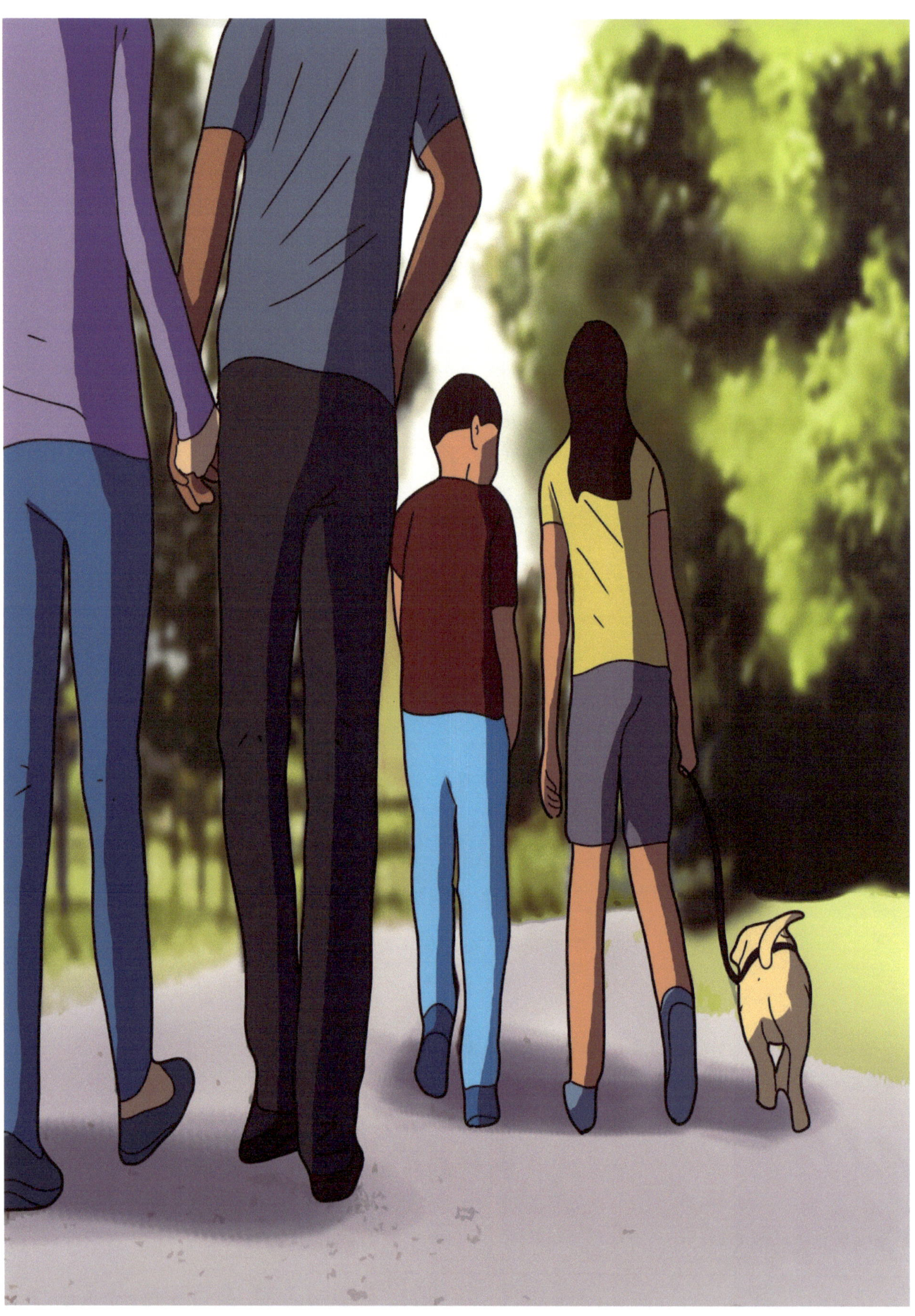

The next day, Mom suggests the family
go for a long walk on a local park trail.
Ali and Ky are very excited to walk and
get some fresh air.
The walking trail is 3 miles long, which is
plenty of time for Ali and Ky to get out
of the house and enjoy the outdoors.
During the walk, Ali and Ky spend time
talking to Mom and Dad, and also laughing
about some of their favorite books and
movies.
Mom suggests they pick up takeout for
dinner from their favorite restaurant.
"Hooray!" say Ali and Ky.
Ali and Ky miss having dinner from their
favorite restaurant.
Ali ordered Chicken fingers and French
fries, while Ky had pasta with tomato
sauce.
"Yum Yum, this is delicious!" cheer Ali
and Ky.

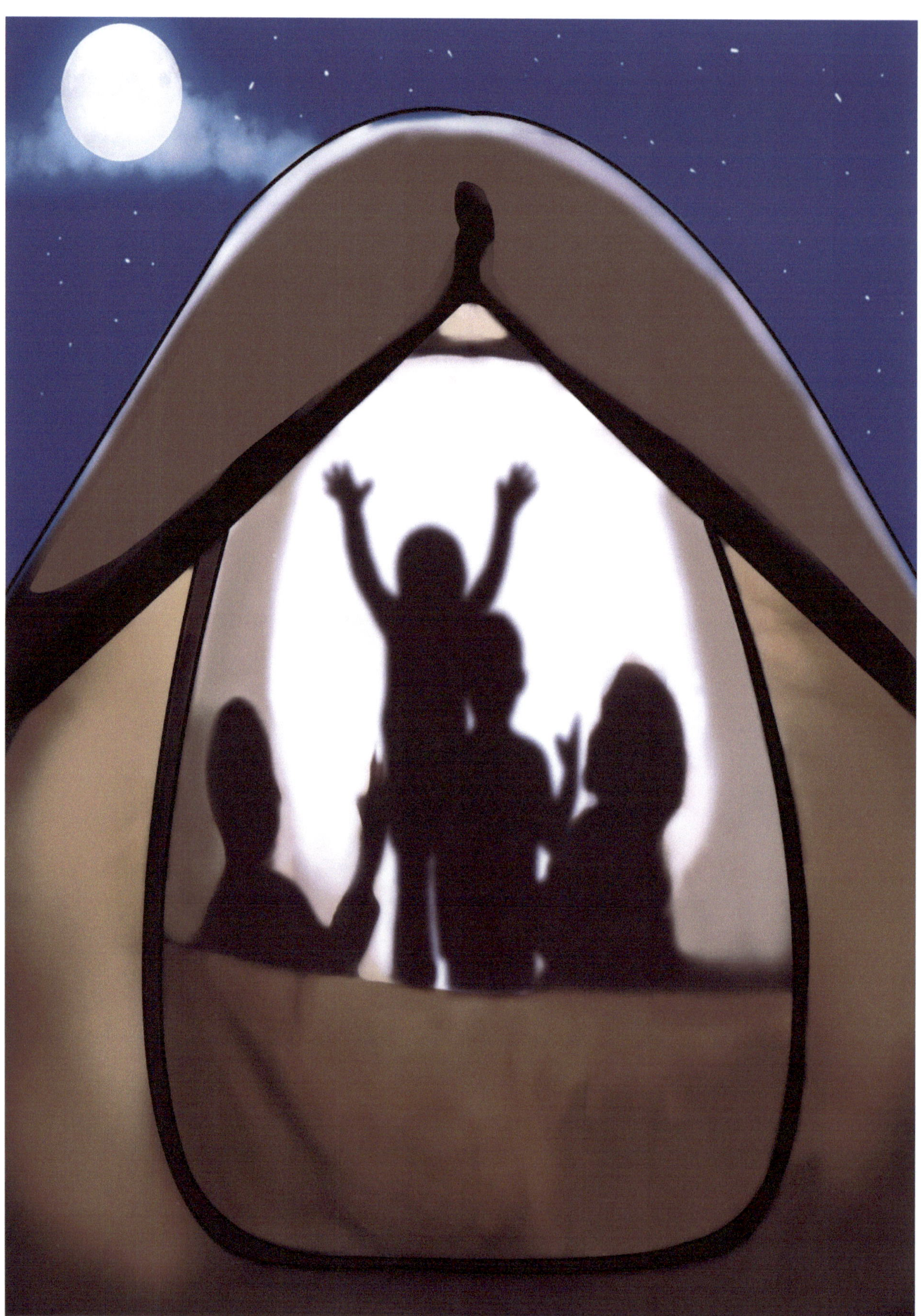

The next day, "Mom, what is there to
do?" asks Ali.

"Yeah, I'm bored, there is nothing to
do," says Ky.

"There is plenty to do" says Mom.
"Tonight we are going to camp in the
backyard with tents, sleeping bags,
blankets, flash lights, and popcorn,"
says Mom.

"Yeah and we can tell scary stories!"
says Ali excitedly.
"Yeah and we can eat S'mores!" says
Ky.

Ali and Ky love to camp, tell scary
stories and eat Smores.

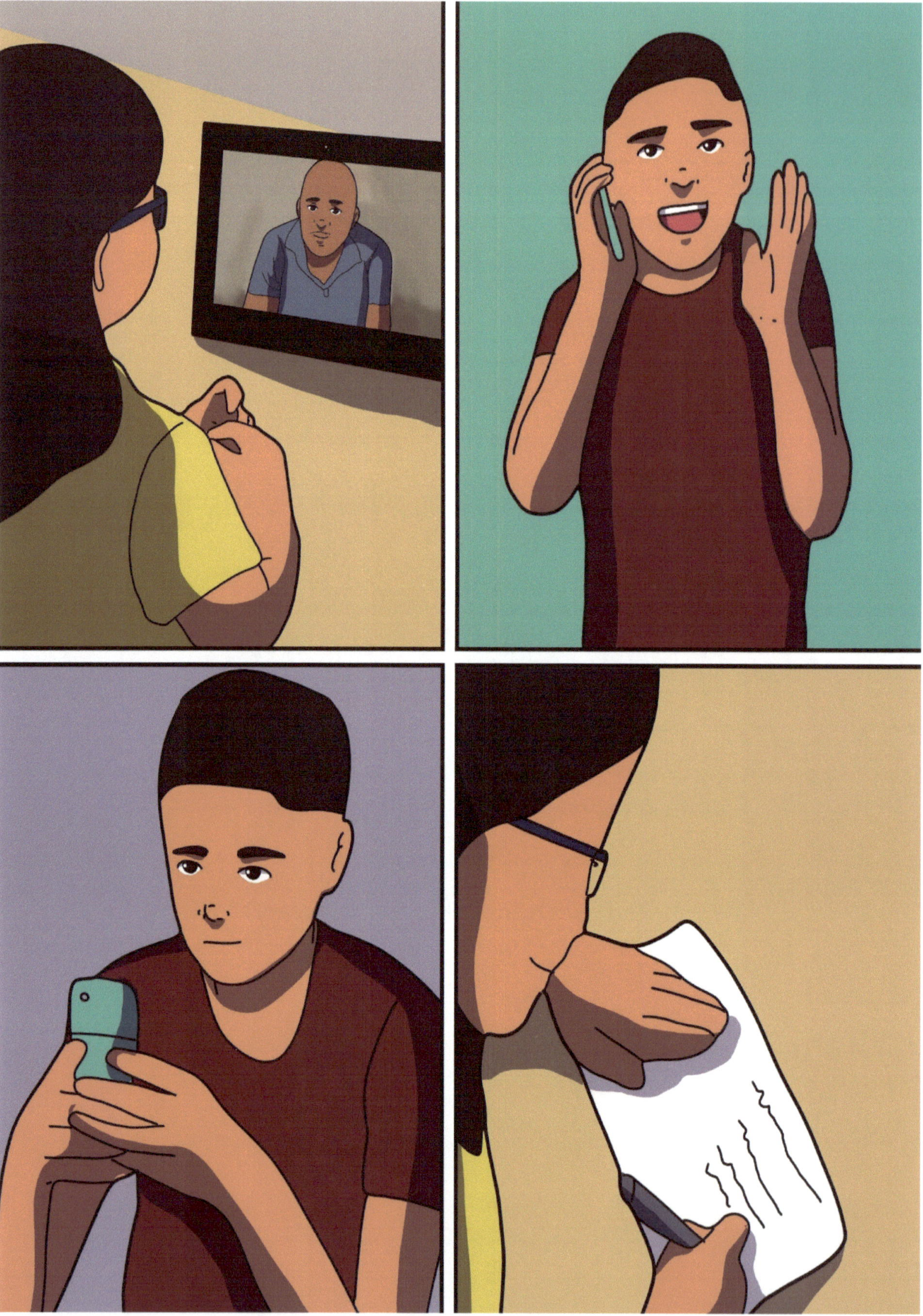

The next day, "Dad, we miss our family
and friends. Can we go for a visit?"
asks Ali and Ky.
"We cannot go for a visit due to the
quarantine but here are a number of
ways we can connect and see how
they are doing." says Dad

Here are a few suggestions to stay
connected:

Video or Instant Message

Call

Text message

Write a letter

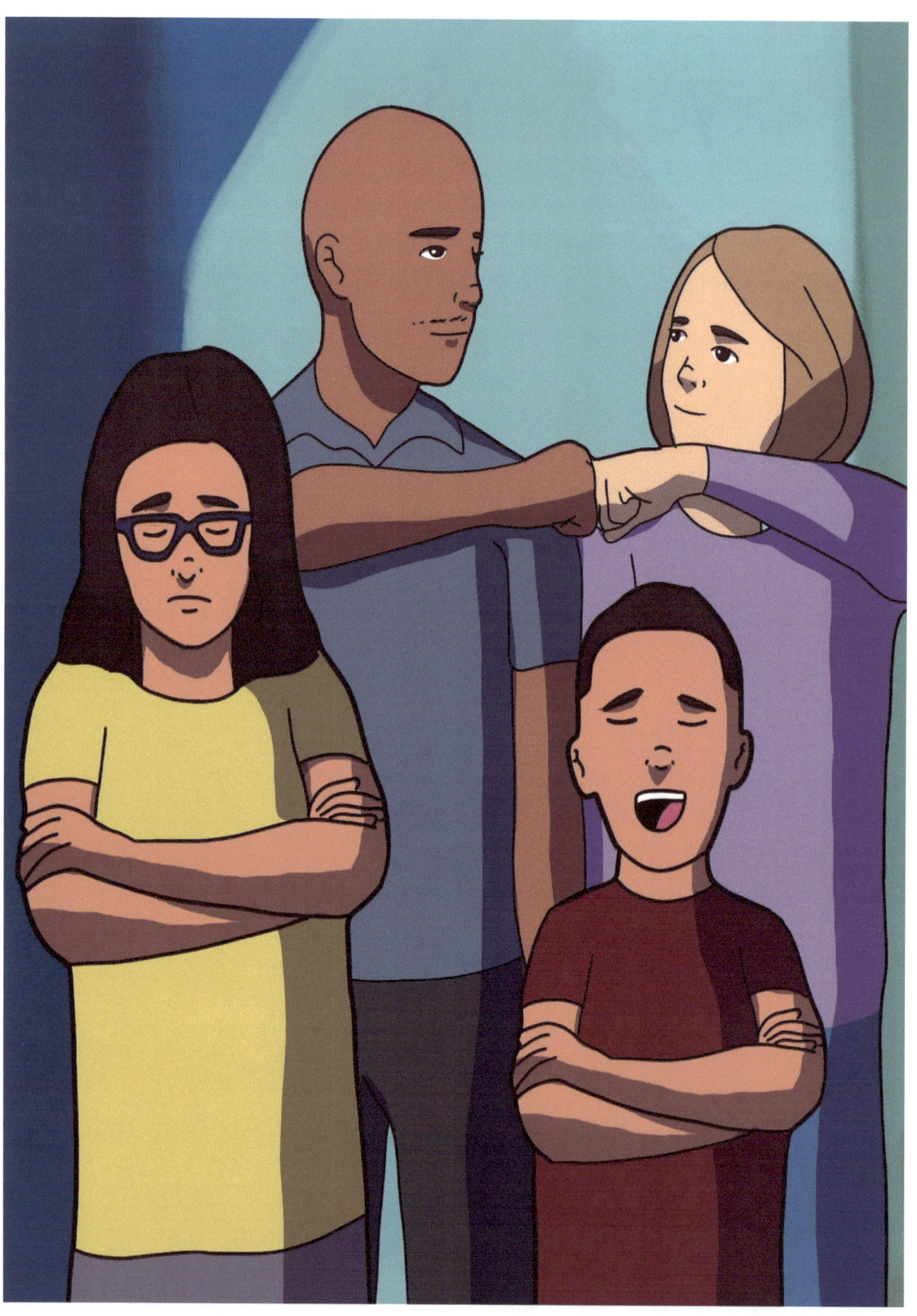

The next day "Mom, can we do something?" asks Ali. "Yeah, I'm bored, there is nothing to do," says Ky.

"There is plenty to do" says Mom.

"You can read a book, do a homework assignment, or play a board game," says Mom.

"You can clean your room, we can paint the basement, or clean out the garage," says Dad.

"You can feed the dog, vacuum the rugs, sweep, and mop the floors," says Dad.

Ali and Ky look at each other and say "No thanks! We will find something to do!" Mom and Dad look at each other, laugh, and say "works every time!"

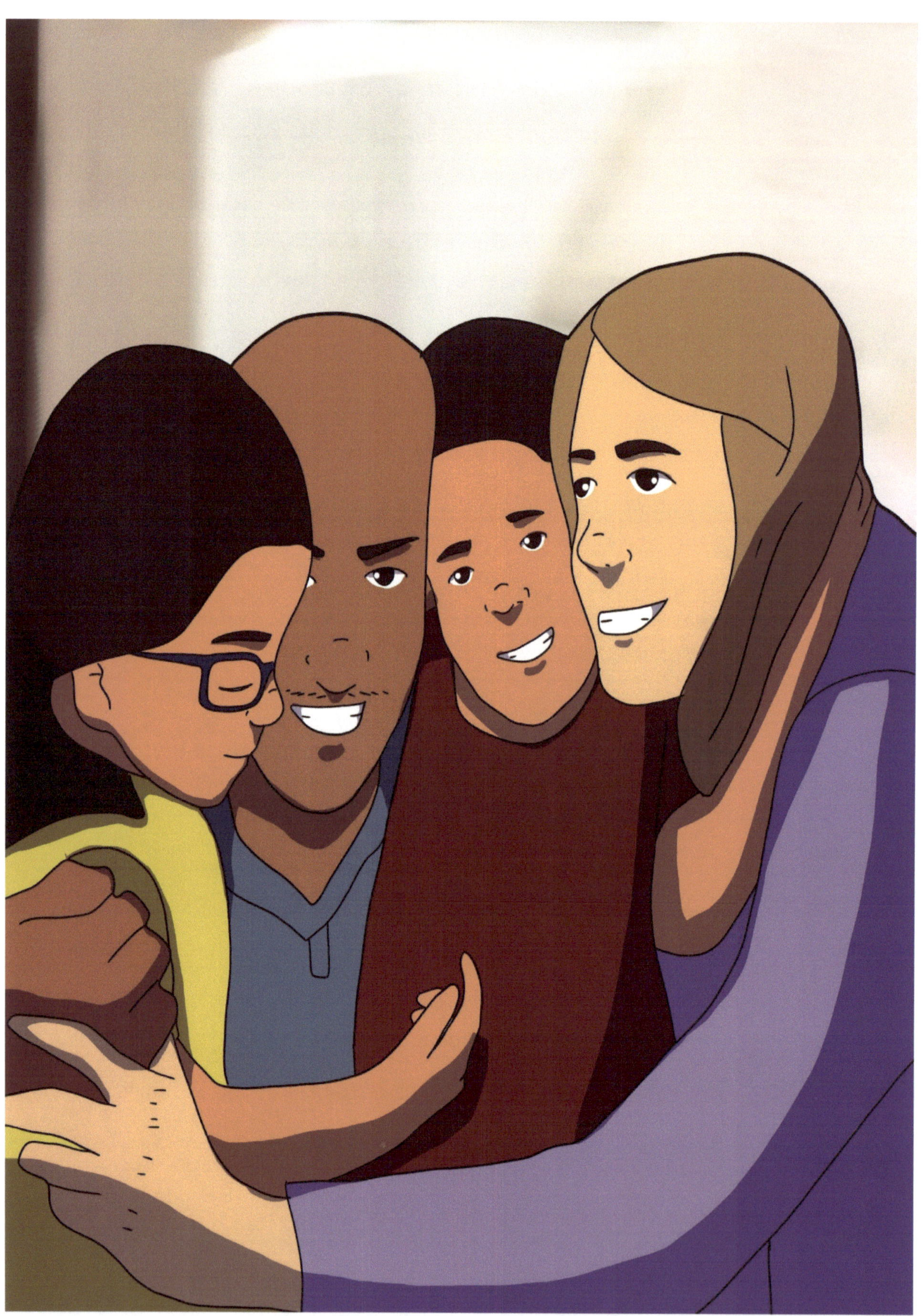

The next day, "How long will we have
to deal with the Coronavirus?" asks
Ali.

"Yeah, how long?" asks Ky.

"We are not sure right now, but we
know we are going to get through
this," says Mom

"And we are going to do it together as
a family," reassures Dad.

"Family Hug!" says Dad as he squeezes
them all together.

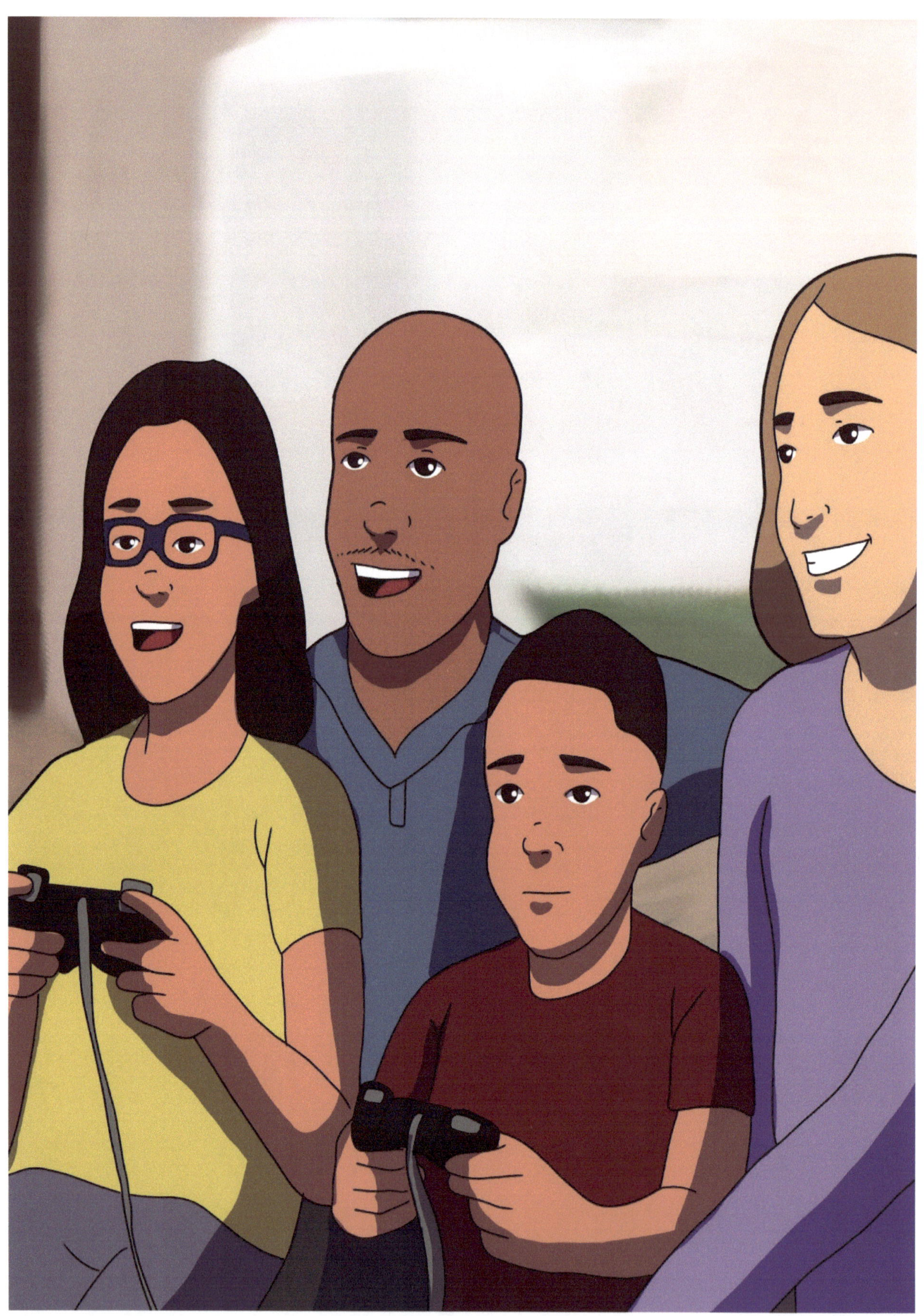

The Coronavirus has impacted and affected the world in many different ways. Even though we are dealing with the Coronavirus quarantine, we are fortunate that this has become a time for our family to press the reset button and reconnect with one another. It has helped us to reprioritize and place value on the things that matter the most, family. These are just a few light hearted ways our family has persevered through the Coronavirus pandemic and social distancing.

Our thoughts and prayers are with all of the families who have been impacted by the COVID-19 (Coronavirus). Please stay safe, healthy, and help one another.